Female Bodybuilding Myths and Facts

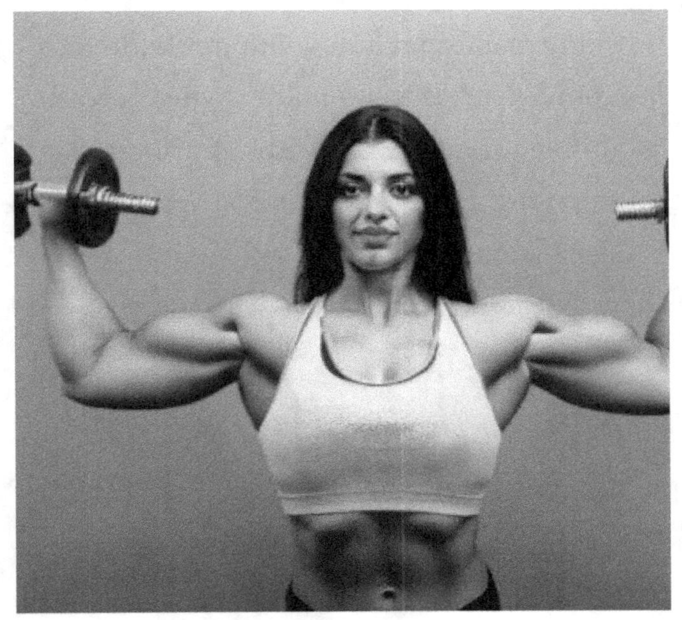

Debunking the Misconceptions About This Sport

Jade Green

Table of Contents

Introduction

Welcome to "Female Bodybuilding Myths and Facts: Debunking the Misconceptions About This Sport." In recent years, female bodybuilding has gained significant attention and popularity as women across the globe have embraced the pursuit of strength, muscle development, and physical empowerment. However, along with its growing popularity, numerous myths and misconceptions have arisen, often overshadowing the true essence and benefits of this sport.

This book aims to dispel the myths surrounding female bodybuilding and provide factual information to help you gain a comprehensive understanding of this empowering discipline. Whether you are a beginner curious about starting your bodybuilding journey or someone seeking to challenge the prevailing stereotypes, this book will equip you with the knowledge and insights needed to navigate through the sea of misinformation.

Through a combination of scientific research, expert perspectives, and personal experiences, we will explore the multifaceted aspects of female bodybuilding. From addressing common misconceptions about appearance and health to examining the training methods, nutrition, and mental well-being, this book will serve as a comprehensive guide to separate fact from fiction.

We will delve into the historical evolution of female bodybuilding, understanding its roots and the transformative changes it has undergone. Furthermore, we will explore the physical and mental benefits that this sport offers, breaking down the barriers and stereotypes that have limited its recognition and acceptance.

By debunking the prevailing myths, we aim to encourage women to embrace their strength, celebrate their bodies, and challenge societal norms. Female bodybuilding is not solely about aesthetics or conforming to a predefined ideal; it is about reclaiming ownership of one's body, fostering resilience, and cultivating a sense of self-empowerment.

Throughout this book, we will provide practical guidance on training techniques, optimal nutrition, mental fortitude, and the impact of female bodybuilding on overall health and well-being. Our goal is to empower you with the knowledge and tools necessary to embark on your own bodybuilding journey, shatter the myths that surround it, and embrace the transformative power of this sport.

Chapter 1

Understanding Female Bodybuilding

The Evolution of Female Bodybuilding

Female bodybuilding has come a long way since its inception, evolving from a niche activity to a recognized sport that celebrates women's strength, dedication, and physical prowess. In this chapter, we will explore the fascinating journey of female bodybuilding, tracing its roots and examining the pivotal moments that have shaped it into what it is today.

The history of female bodybuilding can be traced back to the early 20th century when strongwomen like Katie Sandwina and Abbye "Pudgy" Stockton emerged as symbols of female strength and power. These pioneering women defied societal norms by showcasing their muscular physiques and demonstrating exceptional physical abilities.

However, it was not until the 1970s that female bodybuilding gained significant attention and began to establish itself as a legitimate sport. The iconic figures of that era, such as Rachel McLish and Lisa Lyon, inspired countless women to embrace weightlifting and reshape their bodies. The emergence of competitions specifically for female bodybuilders, such as the Miss Olympia contest, provided a platform for these women to showcase their hard work and dedication.

Over the years, female bodybuilding has faced its share of challenges and controversies. As the sport gained popularity, the prevailing societal notions of femininity clashed with the muscular physiques of female bodybuilders. Criticism and scrutiny regarding their appearance and the potential loss of traditional femininity became pervasive.

Nevertheless, female bodybuilders persisted and continued to push the boundaries, challenging the existing stereotypes and showcasing the incredible results of their disciplined training and nutrition regimens. With the passage of time, the perception of female bodybuilding gradually shifted, and the focus began to shift from aesthetics alone to the celebration of strength, athleticism, and the remarkable dedication of these women.

In this chapter, we will delve into the key moments and influential figures who have shaped the evolution of female bodybuilding. We will examine the challenges faced by early pioneers and the impact they had on breaking down barriers for future generations. By understanding the history of female bodybuilding, we can gain a deeper appreciation for the journey that has led us to the present day.

As we explore the evolution of female bodybuilding, we will also discuss how the sport has diversified and expanded, offering different categories and divisions to accommodate a wider range of physiques and goals. This inclusivity has allowed women from various backgrounds and with different body types to participate in the sport and find their own unique path within it.

Understanding the evolution of female bodybuilding is crucial to appreciate the progress made and the challenges that still lie ahead. By recognizing the struggles and triumphs of those who paved the way, we can celebrate the current state of female bodybuilding and work towards a future that embraces diversity, empowers women, and shatters any remaining misconceptions about this empowering sport.

The Benefits of Female Bodybuilding

Female bodybuilding is not just about building muscle and sculpting an impressive physique; it offers a multitude of benefits that extend beyond the physical realm. In this section, we will explore the wide-ranging advantages that female bodybuilding brings to the lives of women who choose to participate in this empowering sport.

1. Increased Strength and Physical Fitness: Engaging in regular weightlifting and resistance training promotes significant increases in strength, endurance, and overall physical fitness. By challenging their muscles through targeted exercises, female bodybuilders develop functional strength that enhances their daily activities and promotes longevity.

2. Enhanced Body Composition: Contrary to popular misconceptions, female bodybuilding does not automatically lead to bulky or masculine physiques. Instead, it allows women to sculpt their bodies, develop lean muscle mass, and reduce body fat, resulting in a toned and athletic appearance. Bodybuilding provides the opportunity to shape one's physique according to personal goals and preferences.

3. *Improved Bone Density and Joint Health:* Weight-bearing exercises, which are integral to female bodybuilding, stimulate bone remodeling and help increase bone mineral density. This is especially important for women, as they are more susceptible to conditions like osteoporosis. Additionally, strength training helps improve joint stability and reduce the risk of injuries.

4. *Metabolic Boost and Weight Management:* Building and maintaining muscle mass is essential for a healthy metabolism. The increased muscle mass developed through bodybuilding raises the basal metabolic rate, which means the body burns more calories at rest. This can aid in weight management and contribute to long-term fat loss.

5. *Mental and Emotional Well-being:* Female bodybuilding goes beyond physical transformation; it has a profound impact on mental and emotional well-being. Engaging in regular exercise releases endorphins, which promote a positive mood and reduce stress and anxiety. Additionally, bodybuilding instills discipline, perseverance, and a sense of accomplishment, boosting self-confidence and self-esteem.

*6. **Empowerment and Body Positivity:*** Female bodybuilding allows women to challenge societal expectations and redefine beauty standards. By embracing their strength and muscularity, female bodybuilders reclaim ownership of their bodies and celebrate their unique physical attributes. This promotes body positivity and empowers women to appreciate their strength, resilience, and inherent beauty in diverse forms.

*7. **Sense of Community and Support:*** The female bodybuilding community offers a supportive network of like-minded individuals who share a passion for fitness, strength, and self-improvement. Connecting with fellow female bodybuilders provides inspiration, camaraderie, and a sense of belonging, which can contribute to overall motivation and personal growth.

*8. **Setting and Achieving Goals:*** Bodybuilding is a goal-oriented pursuit that requires dedication, discipline, and continuous self-improvement. By setting specific training and nutrition goals, female bodybuilders develop a focused mindset and learn the value of perseverance and hard work. Achieving these goals, whether they are related to strength, physique, or competition, fosters a sense of accomplishment and personal growth.

The Role of Nutrition in Female Bodybuilding

Nutrition plays a vital role in the success of female bodybuilders. Fueling the body with the right nutrients is essential for muscle growth, performance, and overall health. In this section, we will explore the significance of nutrition in female bodybuilding and discuss key considerations for optimal dietary support.

1. Macronutrients: Protein, carbohydrates, and fats are the three macronutrients that form the foundation of a balanced diet for female bodybuilders. Protein is crucial for muscle repair and growth, while carbohydrates provide energy for workouts and replenish glycogen stores. Healthy fats support hormone production, joint health, and overall well-being. Balancing macronutrient intake based on individual goals and training requirements is key to optimizing performance and physique.

2. Caloric Intake: Determining the appropriate caloric intake is essential for female bodybuilders. Whether the goal is building muscle or losing body fat, maintaining a caloric balance that aligns with the desired outcome is crucial. Calculating daily caloric needs based on factors such as basal metabolic rate, activity level, and specific goals helps female bodybuilders stay on track and achieve their desired body composition.

3. *Meal Timing and Frequency:* The timing and frequency of meals can impact energy levels, muscle recovery, and nutrient utilization. Some female bodybuilders find success with traditional three meals a day, while others prefer to divide their caloric intake into smaller, more frequent meals. Meal timing around workouts, ensuring pre- and post-workout nutrition, can enhance performance and recovery. Finding a meal schedule that works best for individual needs and preferences is essential.

4. *Micronutrients and Supplements:* In addition to macronutrients, micronutrients, such as vitamins and minerals, are vital for overall health and well-being. Ensuring an adequate intake of essential micronutrients through a varied and balanced diet supports optimal body function. Additionally, targeted supplementation may be beneficial to fill any nutritional gaps or support specific needs, although it is important to consult with a healthcare professional or registered dietitian before incorporating supplements.

5. *Hydration:* Staying properly hydrated is crucial for female bodybuilders. Water is involved in various physiological processes, including digestion, nutrient absorption, and muscle function. Adequate hydration supports optimal performance, muscle recovery, and overall health. Female bodybuilders should strive to drink enough water throughout the day, especially during workouts and in hot environments.

6. *Individualization and Tracking:* Every female bodybuilder is unique, with different training goals, body compositions, and dietary preferences. It is important to personalize nutrition strategies based on individual needs, monitor progress, and make adjustments as necessary. Tracking food intake, body measurements, and performance metrics can provide valuable insights and guide adjustments to optimize results.

Understanding the role of nutrition in female bodybuilding empowers women to make informed choices that support their goals and overall well-being. By prioritizing proper nutrition, female bodybuilders can maximize their potential, enhance performance, and achieve the desired physique. In the following chapters, we will delve deeper into specific nutrition strategies, meal planning, and supplementation to provide practical guidance for female bodybuilders on their journey to success.

Common Misconceptions and Stereotypes

Female bodybuilding has long been plagued by numerous misconceptions and stereotypes that often overshadow the reality of this empowering sport. In this section, we will address some of the most prevalent misconceptions and challenge the stereotypes surrounding female bodybuilders.

1. Myth: Female Bodybuilders Become Masculine - One of the most enduring myths surrounding female bodybuilding is the belief that engaging in weightlifting and building muscle will automatically result in a masculine appearance. In reality, the muscularity of female bodybuilders is a product of dedicated training, specific nutrition, and genetic factors. It is important to understand that each woman's physique will respond differently to training and that achieving a "bulky" appearance requires years of intentional effort, specialized training, and often the use of performance-enhancing substances.

2. Myth: Female Bodybuilders are Unhealthy - Another common misconception is that female bodybuilders are inherently unhealthy due to their muscular physiques and intensive training routines. However, when approached with proper knowledge and a balanced approach to training and nutrition, female bodybuilding can be a path to improved health and well-being. Many female bodybuilders prioritize overall health by focusing on balanced nutrition, cardiovascular fitness, and monitoring their body's response to training.

3. Myth: Female Bodybuilding is Only for Professional Athletes - Female bodybuilding is often mistakenly assumed to be a pursuit exclusively for professional athletes or competitors. In reality, bodybuilding can be a personal journey for any woman seeking to improve her strength, fitness, and self-confidence. It offers a platform for self-expression, personal growth, and a way to celebrate and embrace one's physical capabilities.

4. Myth: Female Bodybuilders Always Use Steroids - While the use of performance-enhancing substances is a concern in various sports, it is important to recognize that not all female bodybuilders use steroids or other banned substances. The dedication, discipline, and consistent training of natural female bodybuilders can produce remarkable results without the aid of performance-enhancing drugs. It is crucial to differentiate between those who engage in drug-free bodybuilding and those who may use substances, as the motivations, goals, and approaches may differ significantly.

5. Myth: Female Bodybuilding Negatively Affects Fertility - Concerns about fertility and reproductive health often arise when discussing female bodybuilding. However, with proper nutrition, training, and an overall healthy lifestyle, female bodybuilding does not inherently impact fertility. Women can engage in bodybuilding while maintaining regular menstrual cycles and healthy reproductive functions. It is essential to approach bodybuilding with a balanced perspective and consult with healthcare professionals regarding any concerns related to fertility.

Challenging these misconceptions and stereotypes surrounding female bodybuilding is crucial for recognizing the true essence and benefits of this empowering sport. By dispelling these myths, we can celebrate the strength, dedication, and achievements of female bodybuilders, fostering a more inclusive and informed understanding of the sport.

As we continue our journey through the world of female bodybuilding, we will further debunk misconceptions, address concerns, and provide evidence-based information to empower women who aspire to participate in this transformative sport. Together, we can dismantle stereotypes and promote a more accurate and empowering narrative surrounding female bodybuilding.

Chapter 2

Debunking Myths About Female Bodybuilders

Myth 1: Female Bodybuilders Become Masculine

One of the persistent and misleading myths surrounding female bodybuilders is the notion that engaging in weightlifting and building muscle will result in a masculinized appearance. This myth not only undermines the achievements and hard work of female bodybuilders but also perpetuates stereotypes that discourage women from embracing their physical strength. In this chapter, we will debunk this myth and shed light on the realities of female bodybuilding.

Contrary to popular belief, female bodybuilders do not automatically develop masculine features simply by engaging in resistance training and building muscle. The development of a highly muscular physique requires a combination of genetic factors, specific training methods, and often the use of performance-enhancing substances, which are not representative of the majority of female bodybuilders.

The muscularity exhibited by professional female bodybuilders on stage is the result of years of focused training, rigorous nutrition plans, and a specific goal to develop significant muscle mass. It is important to recognize that each woman's body will respond differently to training, and the extent to which muscles develop is highly individual.

Moreover, the physique achieved by female bodybuilders is a personal choice and reflects their dedication and commitment to the sport. Many female bodybuilders strive to achieve a balanced, athletic appearance rather than an exaggerated level of muscularity. They prioritize muscle definition, symmetry, and proportion, which are hallmarks of a well-rounded physique.

It is crucial to separate the aesthetic goals pursued by professional bodybuilders from those of recreational or fitness-oriented female bodybuilders. The majority of women who engage in weightlifting and resistance training will develop strength and muscle tone without becoming excessively muscular. Building lean muscle mass not only contributes to a sculpted physique but also offers numerous health benefits, including improved metabolism, increased bone density, and enhanced overall physical fitness.

Furthermore, it is important to recognize that femininity is not defined solely by appearance but encompasses a spectrum of qualities and characteristics that are not limited by physical attributes. Female bodybuilders can be strong, muscular, and feminine simultaneously, as femininity is a personal expression that extends beyond societal expectations.

By debunking the myth that female bodybuilders become masculine, we can celebrate the diversity of women's bodies and challenge narrow definitions of femininity. Female bodybuilders deserve recognition for their hard work, dedication, and achievements in sculpting their physiques according to their personal goals. As we delve deeper into this chapter, we will continue to address other common misconceptions and stereotypes surrounding female bodybuilders, providing evidence-based information to promote a more informed and inclusive understanding of the sport.

Myth 2: Female Bodybuilders are Unhealthy

Another prevalent myth surrounding female bodybuilders is the misconception that they are inherently unhealthy due to their muscular physiques and intensive training routines. This myth undermines the dedication, discipline, and commitment of female bodybuilders and fails to recognize the significant health benefits associated with their lifestyle. In this chapter, we will debunk this myth and shed light on the realities of the health and well-being of female bodybuilders.

Contrary to the misconception, female bodybuilders who approach their training and nutrition with knowledge and balance can achieve remarkable levels of health and well-being. Engaging in regular resistance training, along with a structured nutrition plan, contributes to numerous positive health outcomes for female bodybuilders.

Firstly, female bodybuilding promotes the development of lean muscle mass, which plays a crucial role in overall health. Increased muscle mass helps boost metabolism, as muscles require more energy to maintain than fat tissue. This, in turn, can support healthy weight management and decrease the risk of conditions such as obesity and metabolic disorders.

Secondly, bodybuilding fosters improved bone density. Weight-bearing exercises, which are integral to resistance training, stimulate bone remodeling and strengthen bone structure. This is especially important for women, as they are more prone to conditions like osteoporosis. By engaging in bodybuilding, female athletes can enhance their bone health and reduce the risk of fractures and bone-related issues.

Furthermore, female bodybuilders often prioritize their nutrition to support their training goals and overall well-being. They learn to balance macronutrients, ensuring an adequate intake of protein, carbohydrates, and healthy fats. By meeting their nutritional needs, female bodybuilders provide their bodies with the necessary fuel for workouts, optimal recovery, and overall vitality.

It is essential to recognize that female bodybuilders can also prioritize cardiovascular health alongside their resistance training. Many incorporate cardiovascular exercises into their routines to improve endurance, promote heart health, and enhance overall cardiovascular fitness. This comprehensive approach to training contributes to a well-rounded and healthy lifestyle.

It is worth noting that like any athletic endeavor, female bodybuilding requires careful management to minimize the risk of potential health issues. This includes monitoring training intensity, allowing for proper recovery, and addressing any potential imbalances or injuries. Responsible female bodybuilders work closely with healthcare professionals and coaches to ensure their training and nutrition plans align with their individual needs and goals.

Debunking the myth that female bodybuilders are unhealthy is crucial for recognizing the positive impact this sport can have on overall well-being. By highlighting the health benefits associated with female bodybuilding, we can challenge the misconceptions and celebrate the dedication, discipline, and commitment that female bodybuilders bring to their pursuit of a strong and healthy physique.

As we continue our exploration of female bodybuilding, we will address additional misconceptions and stereotypes, providing evidence-based information to promote a more informed understanding of the sport and its positive impact on the health and well-being of women who embrace this empowering discipline.

Myth 3: Female Bodybuilding is Only for Professional Athletes

A common myth surrounding female bodybuilding is the belief that it is an activity exclusively reserved for professional athletes. This misconception undermines the inclusive nature of the sport and overlooks the countless women who engage in bodybuilding for personal growth, self-improvement, and a variety of fitness goals. In this chapter, we will debunk this myth and shed light on the diverse range of individuals who participate in female bodybuilding.

Female bodybuilding encompasses a broad spectrum of participation, ranging from recreational enthusiasts to competitive athletes. While professional bodybuilding competitions exist, the majority of female bodybuilders engage in the sport as a personal journey of self-expression, strength development, and physical empowerment.

Women from all walks of life can benefit from the discipline, dedication, and sense of accomplishment that bodybuilding offers. It is a journey that transcends age, background, and fitness level. Female bodybuilding allows individuals to set personal goals, challenge their limits, and celebrate their unique progress, regardless of whether they step onto a competition stage.

Many women are drawn to bodybuilding as a means to improve their physical fitness, transform their bodies, and enhance their overall well-being. By engaging in resistance training and focused workouts, women can increase their strength, build lean muscle mass, and improve their body composition. Bodybuilding provides a platform for personal growth, self-confidence, and a deep appreciation of the strength and capabilities of the female body.

Female bodybuilding also offers a supportive community of like-minded individuals who share a passion for fitness, self-improvement, and empowerment. This community welcomes women of all backgrounds and aspirations, fostering an environment where individuals can connect, share experiences, and find inspiration. This inclusive atmosphere promotes personal growth and encourages women to challenge their own limits in a supportive and encouraging space.

It is important to recognize that female bodybuilding is not solely about professional competition. While some women do choose to compete at various levels, many others engage in bodybuilding as a lifestyle choice, embracing the physical and mental benefits it offers. Whether the goal is to build strength, enhance physique, or simply improve overall well-being, female bodybuilding provides a flexible framework that adapts to individual needs and aspirations.

By debunking the myth that female bodybuilding is only for professional athletes, we can celebrate the diverse range of women who engage in this empowering sport. Women of all backgrounds, ages, and fitness levels can find fulfillment, self-improvement, and a sense of community within the world of female bodybuilding.

As we progress through this chapter, we will continue to challenge misconceptions and stereotypes surrounding female bodybuilders, showcasing the multitude of motivations and goals that drive women to embrace this transformative discipline.

Myth 4: Female Bodybuilders Always Use Steroids

A prevalent myth surrounding female bodybuilders is the assumption that they universally rely on steroids or other performance-enhancing substances to achieve their muscular physiques. This misconception undermines the dedication, hard work, and discipline of female bodybuilders while overlooking the significant number of women who engage in the sport naturally. In this chapter, we will debunk this myth and shed light on the reality of drug-free female bodybuilding.

While it is true that some individuals in the world of bodybuilding, both male and female, have chosen to use performance-enhancing substances, it is incorrect to assume that all female bodybuilders fall into this category. The decision to use steroids or other substances is highly individual and varies among athletes within the sport.

In reality, many female bodybuilders choose to compete in natural bodybuilding federations, where the use of performance-enhancing drugs is strictly prohibited. These women dedicate themselves to a drug-free approach, relying solely on their genetics, training, and nutrition to achieve their goals. Natural bodybuilding competitions provide a platform for these athletes to showcase their hard work and achievements without the use of banned substances.

Moreover, even within non-natural bodybuilding federations, not all female competitors use steroids. Many women engage in bodybuilding as a personal journey, focusing on self-improvement, strength development, and overall well-being without resorting to performance-enhancing substances. Their success is a result of discipline, dedication, and consistency in their training and nutrition regimens.

It is important to recognize that female bodybuilders who choose to compete in natural federations or pursue drug-free bodybuilding face unique challenges. They must adhere to strict guidelines and undergo thorough testing to ensure compliance with anti-doping regulations. These women demonstrate that remarkable physiques and athletic achievements can be attained without the use of steroids or other banned substances.

By debunking the myth that all female bodybuilders use steroids, we can acknowledge and celebrate the accomplishments of natural and drug-free female athletes who devote themselves to the sport with integrity and dedication. It is crucial to distinguish between those who choose to use performance-enhancing substances and those who embrace a drug-free approach, as their motivations, goals, and methods may significantly differ.

As we continue our exploration of female bodybuilding, we will provide further insights into the training, nutrition, and mindset of both natural and non-natural bodybuilders. By shedding light on the reality of drug-free female bodybuilding, we aim to promote a more informed and inclusive understanding of the sport and the women who passionately engage in it.

Myth 5: Female Bodybuilding Negatively Affects Fertility

A commonly perpetuated myth surrounding female bodybuilders is the belief that their intense training and muscular physiques have a detrimental effect on fertility. This myth undermines the achievements and dedication of female bodybuilders while instilling unwarranted concerns about reproductive health. In this chapter, we will debunk this myth and explore the realities of female bodybuilding and its impact on fertility.

Engaging in bodybuilding, when approached responsibly and with attention to overall health, does not inherently impede fertility in women. It is important to understand that the human body is resilient and adaptable, capable of maintaining normal physiological functions, including reproductive health, even during periods of intense physical training.

While extreme training regimens and extreme body fat levels can potentially disrupt the menstrual cycle and affect fertility, it is crucial to recognize that such extreme conditions are not representative of the majority of female bodybuilders. Most female bodybuilders maintain a healthy body composition, balanced nutrition, and appropriate training intensity, allowing them to preserve their reproductive functions.

Female bodybuilders who prioritize their overall well-being, including proper nutrition, sufficient rest and recovery, and monitoring their body's response to training, can maintain regular menstrual cycles and healthy reproductive function. Maintaining a balanced approach to training, nutrition, and overall lifestyle is key to ensuring optimal fertility for women engaging in bodybuilding.

It is worth noting that every woman's body is unique, and individual responses to training and lifestyle factors can vary. Some female bodybuilders may experience temporary disruptions in their menstrual cycles, known as exercise-induced amenorrhea, due to factors such as energy imbalance, excessive training volume, or inadequate nutrition. However, these issues are not exclusive to bodybuilding and can occur in various athletic activities.

Importantly, exercise-induced amenorrhea is typically reversible with appropriate modifications to training, nutrition, and lifestyle. Seeking guidance from healthcare professionals, such as gynecologists or sports medicine specialists, can help female bodybuilders manage any potential concerns and ensure optimal reproductive health.

Debunking the myth that female bodybuilding negatively affects fertility is crucial for providing accurate information and alleviating unnecessary concerns. Responsible female bodybuilders who prioritize their overall health, maintain a balanced approach to training, and monitor their bodies' responses can engage in bodybuilding without compromising their fertility.

As we continue to explore the world of female bodybuilding, we will address additional myths and misconceptions, providing evidence-based information to foster a more informed understanding of the sport and its impact on various aspects of women's health.

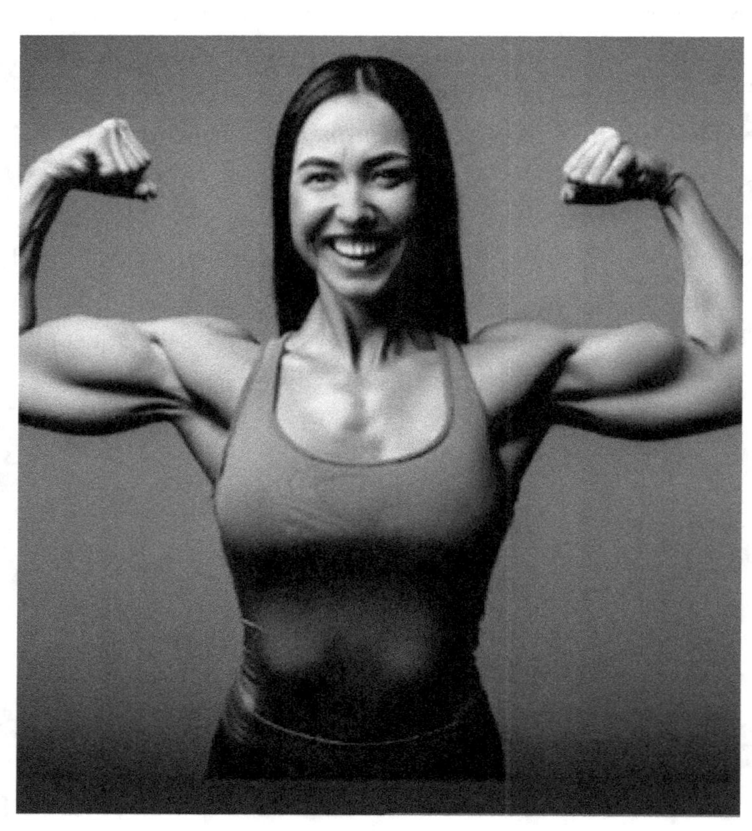

Chapter 3

Training for Female Bodybuilding

Building Muscle and Strength

Building muscle and developing strength are fundamental aspects of female bodybuilding. In this chapter, we will delve into the principles and techniques involved in training for female bodybuilding, highlighting the strategies that enable women to sculpt their bodies, increase muscle mass, and enhance their overall strength.

One of the primary goals in female bodybuilding is hypertrophy, which refers to the increase in muscle size. To achieve this, an effective training program focuses on progressive overload. Progressive overload involves gradually increasing the demands placed on the muscles over time by adjusting variables such as weight, repetitions, sets, and training frequency.

Resistance training forms the core of a female bodybuilder's workout routine. It typically involves using free weights, machines, or bodyweight exercises to target specific muscle groups. Compound exercises, such as squats, deadlifts, bench presses, and overhead presses, are particularly valuable as they engage multiple muscle groups simultaneously, promoting overall strength and muscle development.

Proper form and technique are crucial in maximizing the benefits of resistance training while minimizing the risk of injury. Learning correct lifting techniques and maintaining good posture during exercises is essential. Beginners may benefit from working with a qualified trainer or coach to ensure proper execution of movements and to design a training program tailored to their specific needs and goals.

Variety and progression are essential elements of an effective training regimen. Varying exercises, rep ranges, and training methods can help prevent plateaus and maintain motivation. Periodization, which involves dividing training into distinct phases with varying intensities and focuses, is commonly employed to optimize progress and minimize the risk of overtraining.

Rest and recovery are integral components of any training program. Allowing adequate time for the body to rest and repair is crucial for muscle growth and overall performance. Female bodybuilders should aim for sufficient sleep, incorporate rest days into their training schedule, and consider active recovery strategies such as stretching or low-impact activities to support overall recovery.

Nutrition plays a vital role in supporting muscle growth and recovery. Consuming adequate protein is crucial, as it provides the necessary building blocks for muscle repair and growth. Additionally, a balanced diet with sufficient calories and macronutrients supports energy levels and overall health, enabling optimal performance during workouts.

It is important to note that individual responses to training can vary, and it may take time to find the ideal training program that works best for each individual. Patience, consistency, and a focus on progressive overload are key principles for achieving desired results in female bodybuilding.

As we proceed through this chapter, we will delve further into specific training methodologies, strategies for targeting specific muscle groups, and the importance of proper recovery. By understanding the principles of training for female bodybuilding, women can develop a focused and effective workout routine that enables them to build muscle, increase strength, and achieve their desired physique.

The Importance of Proper Form and Technique

In the pursuit of building muscle and strength, proper form and technique are paramount in female bodybuilding. It is essential to perform exercises correctly to maximize results, minimize the risk of injury, and ensure efficient muscle activation. In this section, we will explore the importance of proper form and technique in training for female bodybuilding.

Performing exercises with proper form involves maintaining the correct body alignment, executing the movement through the intended range of motion, and engaging the target muscles effectively. By maintaining proper form, you can ensure that the desired muscle groups are being appropriately targeted and activated during each exercise.

One of the primary reasons for focusing on proper form is injury prevention. When exercises are performed with incorrect form, stress can be placed on the wrong muscles or joints, increasing the risk of strain, sprain, or other injuries. By adhering to proper form, you can minimize the likelihood of overloading certain areas and prevent unnecessary stress on your body.

Proper form also enables you to optimize muscle engagement and activation. When exercises are performed with correct technique, the intended muscle groups are targeted more effectively, leading to better muscle development and strength gains. This means that by paying attention to form, you can ensure that you are getting the most out of each exercise and maximizing your results.

Learning proper form and technique is crucial, especially when starting a new exercise or using equipment for the first time. Beginners are encouraged to seek guidance from qualified trainers or coaches who can teach them the correct form for various exercises. They can provide valuable feedback, corrections, and modifications to ensure proper execution and help prevent bad habits from forming.

It is important to focus on quality over quantity when it comes to training. While lifting heavier weights or completing more repetitions may seem tempting, sacrificing form to do so can compromise your results and increase the risk of injury. Maintaining proper form, even with lighter weights, ensures that you are effectively targeting the desired muscles and working towards your goals in a safe and sustainable manner.

Developing body awareness is key to maintaining proper form. Paying attention to your body positioning, posture, and movement during each exercise helps you stay connected to the muscles you are targeting. It allows you to make necessary adjustments to ensure optimal form and engagement.

Regular practice and mindful training contribute to the development of proper form and technique over time. As you become more experienced, your body will adapt to the movements and exercises, allowing you to refine your form and execute exercises with greater precision and control.

In conclusion, proper form and technique are essential in female bodybuilding to maximize results, prevent injuries, and effectively target specific muscle groups. By focusing on maintaining correct form, you can optimize muscle engagement, improve strength gains, and minimize the risk of unnecessary strain on your body. As you progress in your training journey, continue to prioritize and refine your form to ensure continued progress and long-term success in female bodybuilding.

Designing an Effective Workout Routine

Designing an effective workout routine is crucial for achieving optimal results in female bodybuilding. A well-structured program ensures balanced muscle development, progression, and sufficient recovery. In this section, we will explore key considerations and guidelines for designing an effective workout routine tailored to the goals and needs of female bodybuilders.

1. Set Clear Goals: Begin by defining your specific goals in female bodybuilding. Whether your focus is on building muscle, increasing strength, improving overall fitness, or preparing for competition, identifying your objectives will guide the design of your workout routine.

2. Target All Major Muscle Groups: A comprehensive workout routine should include exercises that target all major muscle groups of the body. This includes the chest, back, shoulders, biceps, triceps, legs, and core. Incorporating compound exercises that engage multiple muscle groups simultaneously is an efficient way to stimulate overall muscle growth and strength.

3. Select Appropriate Exercises: Choose exercises that align with your goals and abilities. Include a mix of compound exercises (e.g., squats, deadlifts, bench presses) and isolation exercises (e.g., bicep curls, tricep extensions) to effectively target specific muscles. Consider variations and modifications based on equipment availability, training experience, and individual preferences.

4. *Determine Training Frequency:* Decide on the number of training sessions per week based on your schedule, recovery capacity, and goals. Aim for a balance between training volume and recovery to avoid overtraining. Beginners may start with 2-3 weekly sessions, gradually progressing to 4-5 sessions as their fitness levels and recovery abilities improve.

5. *Plan Progressive Overload:* Incorporate progressive overload into your workout routine to continuously challenge your muscles and promote growth. Gradually increase the intensity, load, repetitions, or training volume over time. This can be achieved by adjusting weights, sets, reps, rest periods, or incorporating advanced training techniques like supersets or drop sets.

6. *Consider Training Split:* Divide your workouts into different training splits to target specific muscle groups on different days. Common training splits include full-body workouts, upper/lower body splits, or dividing workouts by muscle groups (e.g., push/pull/legs). Select a training split that aligns with your goals, time availability, and recovery capabilities.

7. *Incorporate Rest and Recovery:* Allow adequate time for rest and recovery between training sessions. Rest days are essential for muscle repair, growth, and overall performance improvement. Listen to your body, ensure sufficient sleep, and consider implementing active recovery techniques such as stretching, foam rolling, or low-impact cardio activities.

8. *Adjust Based on Progress:* Regularly assess your progress and make necessary adjustments to your workout routine. Track your performance, strength gains, and overall physique changes to identify areas for improvement. Modify exercises, training volume, or intensity as needed to continue challenging your muscles and avoiding plateauing.

9. *Seek Professional Guidance:* If you're new to bodybuilding or require guidance, consider working with a qualified trainer or coach. They can provide expertise in exercise selection, form correction, progression planning, and personalized programming tailored to your goals and abilities.

Overcoming Challenges and Plateaus

In the journey of female bodybuilding, it is common to encounter challenges and plateaus that can hinder progress. Overcoming these obstacles is crucial to maintain motivation, stimulate muscle growth, and continue making advancements in strength and physique. In this section, we will explore strategies to overcome challenges and break through plateaus in female bodybuilding.

1. Reassess Your Goals: Take a moment to reassess your goals and make sure they align with your current aspirations and priorities. Revisiting your objectives can reignite your motivation and provide a fresh perspective on your training journey.

2. Vary Your Training Routine: Plateaus can often occur when the body becomes accustomed to the same training stimulus. Introduce variety into your workout routine by changing exercises, rep ranges, rest periods, or training techniques. This challenges your muscles in new ways, stimulating growth and preventing stagnation.

3. Modify Training Intensity: Adjusting the intensity of your workouts can help overcome plateaus. Incorporate techniques such as drop sets, supersets, or pyramid sets to increase the challenge on your muscles. Additionally, you can manipulate training variables like weights, repetitions, or time under tension to promote adaptation and progress.

4. *Periodize Your Training:* Implementing a periodization strategy in your training program can help overcome plateaus by varying the training stimulus over time. Dividing your training into distinct phases, such as hypertrophy, strength, and endurance, allows for targeted adaptation and prevents the body from adapting to a single stimulus.

5. *Focus on Progressive Overload:* Continuously challenging your muscles through progressive overload is crucial to promote growth and overcome plateaus. Gradually increase the intensity, load, or volume of your training sessions to provide a constant stimulus for improvement.

6. *Prioritize Recovery:* Plateaus can sometimes be a result of insufficient recovery. Ensure you are allowing your body enough time to rest and repair between workouts. Prioritize quality sleep, incorporate active recovery strategies like stretching or foam rolling, and consider deloading weeks or periods of reduced intensity to facilitate recovery.

7. *Fine-Tune Your Nutrition:* Assess your nutrition plan to ensure you are fueling your body appropriately. Adequate protein intake is crucial for muscle growth and recovery. Consider consulting with a registered dietitian to ensure your nutrition supports your training goals and addresses any potential nutrient deficiencies.

8. *Monitor and Track Progress:* Keep a record of your training sessions, including weights used, sets, and repetitions performed. Monitoring your progress allows you to track improvements over time and identify areas for adjustment or improvement.

9. *Stay Motivated and Mentally Engaged:* Plateaus can be mentally challenging, but it is important to stay motivated and focused on your long-term goals. Seek inspiration from other athletes, join a supportive community, or set mini-goals to keep your enthusiasm high.

10. *Seek Professional Guidance:* If you find yourself struggling to overcome challenges or break through plateaus, consider seeking guidance from a qualified trainer or coach. They can provide expert advice, evaluate your training program, and suggest adjustments or advanced techniques to help you move past obstacles.

Chapter 4

Nutrition and Diet for Female Bodybuilders

Understanding Caloric Needs and Macronutrients

Proper nutrition and diet are vital components of female bodybuilding, supporting muscle growth, recovery, and overall performance. In this chapter, we will explore the importance of understanding caloric needs and macronutrients in fueling and optimizing the female bodybuilding journey.

1. Caloric Needs: Understanding your caloric needs is crucial for providing your body with the energy it requires to support training and muscle growth. Caloric needs vary depending on factors such as body composition, metabolism, activity level, and goals. Calculating your Total Daily Energy Expenditure (TDEE) can help determine an appropriate caloric intake.

2. Energy Balance: Achieving the right energy balance is essential. To build muscle, a slight caloric surplus is often required, while fat loss generally necessitates a caloric deficit. It is important to strike a balance that aligns with your goals while ensuring adequate nutrition for optimal health and performance.

3. Macronutrients: Macronutrients, consisting of proteins, carbohydrates, and fats, are the primary sources of energy for the body. Understanding their roles and appropriate intake is essential for female bodybuilders.

- Proteins: Protein is crucial for muscle repair, growth, and maintenance. Aim to consume sufficient protein to support your training goals. Recommendations typically range from 0.8 to 1.2 grams of protein per pound of body weight per day, depending on individual factors and training intensity.

- Carbohydrates: Carbohydrates are the body's primary source of energy, particularly during intense workouts. Consuming adequate carbohydrates provides the fuel necessary to power through training sessions and replenish glycogen stores. Choose complex carbohydrates such as whole grains, fruits, and vegetables for sustained energy.

- Fats: Healthy fats are important for hormone production, joint health, and overall well-being. Include sources of unsaturated fats like avocados, nuts, seeds, and fatty fish in your diet. Aim for a moderate fat intake,

typically around 20-30% of your total daily caloric intake.

4. Meal Timing and Frequency: While meal timing and frequency can be individualized, it is generally beneficial to distribute meals evenly throughout the day. This promotes a steady supply of nutrients for muscle recovery and growth. Some individuals may prefer multiple smaller meals, while others may opt for a few larger meals. Find an approach that suits your preferences and supports your training and energy needs.

5. Micronutrients: In addition to macronutrients, ensure an adequate intake of micronutrients—vitamins, minerals, and antioxidants—through a balanced diet. These nutrients support overall health, immune function, and optimize training adaptations. Include a variety of fruits, vegetables, whole grains, lean proteins, and healthy fats to meet your micronutrient needs.

6. Hydration: Staying adequately hydrated is crucial for optimal performance. Aim to consume water throughout the day, especially before, during, and after workouts. Individual hydration needs vary, so pay attention to your body's signals and adjust water intake accordingly.

7. Supplementation: While a well-rounded diet should provide most of your nutritional needs, some female bodybuilders may benefit from certain supplements. Consult with a healthcare professional or registered dietitian to determine if any specific supplements are necessary based on your individual circumstances.

Remember that nutritional needs are highly individual, and it is important to listen to your body's cues and adapt your diet accordingly. Working with a registered dietitian who specializes in sports nutrition can provide personalized guidance and help tailor your nutrition plan to support your bodybuilding goals.

As we progress through this chapter, we will delve deeper into specific nutrition strategies, meal planning, nutrient timing, and strategies for optimizing performance and recovery. By understanding and implementing proper nutrition and diet principles, you can fuel your body effectively and enhance your progress in female bodybuilding.

The Role of Protein in Muscle Building

Protein plays a vital role in muscle building and is of great importance to female bodybuilders. Understanding its significance and incorporating an adequate protein intake into your diet can support muscle growth, repair, and recovery. In this section, we will explore the role of protein and its impact on the female bodybuilding journey.

Protein serves as the building blocks for muscle tissue. When engaging in resistance training, the muscles undergo microscopic damage. Protein consumption provides the essential amino acids necessary for repairing and rebuilding these muscle fibers, promoting muscle growth and strength development.

1. Muscle Repair and Growth: Protein is crucial for repairing damaged muscle tissue and stimulating muscle protein synthesis, the process by which new muscle proteins are created. Consuming adequate protein allows the body to rebuild and strengthen muscles, leading to improved muscle size, definition, and overall muscularity.

2. Essential Amino Acids: Proteins are made up of amino acids, and certain amino acids are considered essential, meaning the body cannot produce them on its own and must obtain them through the diet. Consuming a variety of protein sources ensures an adequate supply of essential amino acids for muscle protein synthesis.

3. *Protein Quality and Sources:* Different protein sources vary in their amino acid profiles and digestibility. Animal-based sources such as lean meats, poultry, fish, eggs, and dairy products are considered complete proteins, as they provide all essential amino acids in sufficient quantities. Plant-based protein sources like legumes, tofu, tempeh, and quinoa can be combined to create complete protein profiles.

4. *Protein Timing and Distribution:* While total protein intake throughout the day is important, distributing protein intake evenly across meals has shown benefits for muscle protein synthesis. Aim to consume a source of protein with each meal and snack to ensure a steady supply of amino acids for muscle repair and growth.

5. *Protein Recommendations:* Protein needs for female bodybuilders can vary based on factors such as training intensity, body weight, and goals. Recommendations typically range from 0.8 to 1.2 grams of protein per pound of body weight per day. Individual protein requirements may vary, so it is important to listen to your body and adjust your intake based on your specific needs.

6. *Combining Protein and Carbohydrates:* Combining protein with carbohydrates post-workout can enhance muscle recovery and replenish glycogen stores. The carbohydrates help shuttle amino acids into the muscles and promote glycogen synthesis, providing energy for future workouts.

7. *Whole Foods vs. Supplements:* While whole food sources are generally recommended for meeting protein needs, protein supplements such as whey protein, casein protein, or plant-based protein powders can be convenient options to supplement dietary protein intake. However, it is important to prioritize whole foods as the primary source of nutrients whenever possible.

Remember that protein is just one component of a well-rounded diet, and a balanced approach to nutrition is key. Incorporate a variety of protein sources into your meals, including lean meats, poultry, fish, dairy products, legumes, and plant-based proteins. By ensuring an adequate protein intake, you can support muscle building, recovery, and overall progress in female bodybuilding.

Proper Supplementation for Female Bodybuilders

Supplements can be a helpful addition to the diet of female bodybuilders, providing support for specific nutritional needs and enhancing overall performance and recovery. However, it is important to approach supplementation with knowledge and caution. In this section, we will explore proper supplementation for female bodybuilders and highlight key considerations.

1. Individual Needs: Recognize that supplement needs vary among individuals based on factors such as training intensity, goals, dietary preferences, and overall health. What works for one person may not be necessary or suitable for another. Consulting with a healthcare professional or registered dietitian can help determine if supplementation is appropriate for your specific circumstances.

2. Whole Foods First: While supplements can be beneficial, it is important to prioritize whole, nutrient-dense foods as the foundation of your diet. Whole foods provide a wide range of essential nutrients and should form the basis of your nutrition plan. Supplements should complement, not replace, a well-rounded diet.

3. *Protein Supplements:* Protein powders, such as whey protein, casein protein, or plant-based protein powders, can be convenient options for meeting protein needs. They can help ensure an adequate protein intake, especially during periods when whole food sources may be less accessible. Choose high-quality, reputable brands and be mindful of added sugars or unnecessary ingredients.

4. *Essential Nutrients:* Some supplements can help bridge nutrient gaps and support overall health. For example, a multivitamin and mineral supplement can ensure adequate intake of essential vitamins and minerals. Omega-3 fatty acid supplements, derived from sources like fish oil or algae, can provide beneficial fats that support cardiovascular health and inflammation control.

5. *Pre-Workout Supplements:* Pre-workout supplements may contain ingredients like caffeine, creatine, or beta-alanine, which can enhance energy levels, focus, and performance during workouts. However, it is important to be mindful of individual sensitivities and potential side effects. Start with lower doses and assess your response before increasing the intake.

6. *Post-Workout Recovery:* Post-workout supplements can aid in recovery and replenishing nutrients after intense training sessions. Some options include carbohydrate-electrolyte drinks to replenish glycogen stores and promote hydration, as well as branched-chain amino acid (BCAA) supplements to support muscle recovery.

7.   *Personalized Approach:* Understand that supplementation is highly individualized. What works for someone else may not necessarily work for you. Experimenting with supplements should be done cautiously, with attention to how they affect your body, performance, and overall well-being.

8. *Quality and Safety:* When choosing supplements, prioritize quality and safety. Look for reputable brands that undergo third-party testing for purity and label accuracy. Research the ingredients, check for any potential interactions with medications or pre-existing conditions, and follow recommended dosages.

9. *Regular Evaluation:* Regularly reassess your supplement regimen to ensure its relevance and effectiveness. As your goals, training, and overall health evolve, your supplement needs may change. Periodically consult with a healthcare professional or registered dietitian to evaluate and adjust your supplementation as necessary.

Remember that supplements are intended to supplement, not replace, a balanced diet and healthy lifestyle. They should be used judiciously and in conjunction with a well-rounded nutrition plan. Prioritizing whole foods, proper hydration, sufficient sleep, and overall lifestyle factors remain essential for optimal results in female bodybuilding.

As we progress through this chapter, we will delve deeper into specific nutrition strategies, meal planning, and advanced supplementation approaches to provide a comprehensive understanding of fueling your body effectively as a female bodybuilder.

Balancing Diet and Social Life

Maintaining a balanced diet while navigating social events and gatherings is an important aspect of sustainable and enjoyable nutrition for female bodybuilders. Striking a balance between your dietary goals and social life can be challenging, but it is achievable with mindful planning and flexibility. In this section, we will explore strategies for balancing your diet and social life as a female bodybuilder.

1. Plan Ahead: Before attending social events, plan your meals and snacks accordingly. If you know you'll be indulging in a special meal or treat, make adjustments earlier in the day to ensure your overall caloric and nutrient intake remains balanced. Focus on consuming nutrient-dense foods to meet your essential nutritional needs.

2. Communicate Your Goals: Inform your friends, family, and loved ones about your dietary goals and the importance of proper nutrition for your bodybuilding journey. Openly discussing your intentions can help others understand and support your choices, reducing potential pressure or temptation to stray from your diet.

3. Be Mindful of Portions: Enjoy the foods and drinks offered during social events, but be mindful of portion sizes. Practice moderation by selecting smaller servings or sharing dishes with others. This allows you to enjoy the flavors and social aspect while keeping your overall caloric intake in check.

4. *Choose Wisely:* When faced with an array of food options, make conscious choices that align with your dietary goals. Opt for lean protein sources, vegetables, fruits, and whole grains whenever possible. Be selective with indulgent foods or desserts, enjoying them in moderation rather than feeling deprived or completely avoiding them.

5. *Bring Your Own Dish:* If appropriate, offer to bring a dish or contribute to the event's menu. This way, you can ensure there is a nutritious option that aligns with your dietary preferences. Sharing your healthy creations with others can also introduce them to delicious and nutritious alternatives.

6. *Stay Hydrated:* Drinking water throughout social events can help you stay hydrated and feel satiated. It can also prevent overconsumption of high-calorie beverages. If you choose to drink alcohol, do so in moderation and be aware of its caloric content.

7. *Focus on Socializing:* While food plays a significant role in social gatherings, prioritize the social aspect itself. Engage in conversations, connect with others, and enjoy the company of friends and loved ones. Remember that the quality of interactions matters just as much, if not more, than the food being consumed.

8. *Practice Flexible Eating:* Embrace flexibility in your diet to accommodate social occasions. Adopting a flexible eating mindset allows you to enjoy special events without guilt or restriction. Balancing your overall nutrition over time rather than fixating on individual meals or events is key.

9. *Avoid "All or Nothing" Thinking:* It's important to avoid falling into the trap of "all or nothing" thinking when it comes to your diet. One indulgent meal or event does not define your overall progress. Instead of fixating on occasional deviations, focus on consistent adherence to your nutrition plan and long-term goals.

10. *Enjoy the Experience:* Remember that food is not only fuel but also a source of enjoyment and pleasure. Embrace the experience of trying new foods, savoring delicious flavors, and creating lasting memories with loved ones. Balancing your diet and social life means finding joy and satisfaction in both aspects.

Finding a balance between your dietary goals and social life is a personal journey. It may require trial and error, flexibility, and self-compassion. By planning ahead, making mindful choices, and focusing on the overall balance of your nutrition, you can successfully navigate social events while staying on track with your female bodybuilding goals.

As we continue through this chapter, we will explore additional strategies for meal planning, maintaining consistency, and cultivating a positive relationship with food as a female bodybuilder.

Chapter 5

Mental and Emotional Aspects of Female Bodybuilding

Body Image and Self-Esteem

Body image and self-esteem are important psychological aspects of female bodybuilding. Engaging in this sport can have a significant impact on how women perceive themselves and their bodies. In this chapter, we will delve into the complex relationship between body image, self-esteem, and female bodybuilding.

1. Body Image Perception: Female bodybuilders often strive to attain a specific physique through rigorous training and dieting. It is important to recognize that body image perception can vary greatly among individuals. Some may feel empowered and confident with their muscular physiques, while others may experience challenges in accepting and embracing their changing bodies.

*2. **Societal Influences:*** Societal ideals and media portrayals of beauty often emphasize slender and less muscular female bodies. These narrow beauty standards can create unrealistic expectations and put pressure on female bodybuilders to conform to conventional norms. It is crucial to challenge these narrow ideals and celebrate diverse body shapes and sizes.

*3. **Self-Esteem and Body Satisfaction:*** Self-esteem, the overall evaluation of one's self-worth, can be influenced by body image satisfaction. Female bodybuilders may experience fluctuations in self-esteem as they navigate the journey of building and sculpting their bodies. Recognize that self-esteem should be based on a holistic view of oneself, encompassing personal values, achievements, and character, rather than solely on physical appearance.

*4. **Building a Positive Body Image:*** Developing a positive body image involves accepting and appreciating one's body, regardless of societal norms or comparisons to others. Female bodybuilders can cultivate a positive body image by focusing on their strength, physical capabilities, and the overall health benefits of their training. Surrounding oneself with a supportive community and practicing self-compassion are also valuable in promoting a positive body image.

5. *Mental and Emotional Well-Being:* Maintaining mental and emotional well-being is crucial for female bodybuilders. Engaging in self-care practices such as mindfulness, stress management, and relaxation techniques can help manage the pressures and challenges associated with bodybuilding. Prioritizing mental health and seeking support from professionals or support groups can contribute to overall well-being.

6. *Setting Realistic Expectations:* It is important to set realistic expectations and goals in female bodybuilding. Striving for continuous progress while embracing the journey is more sustainable than fixating solely on achieving a specific physique. Celebrate achievements along the way and acknowledge that progress varies individually, emphasizing the importance of self-acceptance and patience.

7. *Healthy Coping Mechanisms:* Female bodybuilding can bring about various emotions and challenges. Adopting healthy coping mechanisms such as seeking social support, engaging in hobbies, practicing mindfulness or journaling, and maintaining a balanced lifestyle can help manage stress and promote emotional well-being.

8. *Embracing Individuality:* Each female bodybuilder is unique, with her own strengths, talents, and qualities that extend beyond her physical appearance. Embrace and celebrate your individuality, focusing on the overall journey of personal growth, self-improvement, and fulfillment.

Remember that body image and self-esteem are deeply personal and can fluctuate throughout the bodybuilding journey. Developing a positive body image and nurturing self-esteem require ongoing self-reflection, self-compassion, and self-acceptance. By prioritizing mental and emotional well-being alongside physical training, female bodybuilders can experience a more holistic and fulfilling approach to the sport.

Dealing with Criticism and Judgment

Engaging in female bodybuilding can subject individuals to criticism and judgment from others who may not understand or appreciate the sport. Dealing with external opinions and navigating societal pressures can be challenging. In this section, we will explore strategies for coping with criticism and judgment as a female bodybuilder.

1. Stay True to Your Goals: Remember your reasons for pursuing female bodybuilding and stay committed to your personal goals. Understand that the opinions of others do not define your journey or your worth. Focus on your own progress, growth, and self-improvement.

2. Educate Others: Take the opportunity to educate others about the sport of female bodybuilding. Share your knowledge, experiences, and the dedication required to pursue this passion. By providing insights and dispelling misconceptions, you can help others gain a better understanding and appreciation for your chosen path.

3. Surround Yourself with Supportive People: Seek out a supportive network of friends, family, and fellow athletes who understand and respect your commitment to female bodybuilding. Surrounding yourself with individuals who appreciate and celebrate your accomplishments can provide encouragement and bolster your confidence in the face of criticism.

4. *Focus on Personal Progress:* Shift your focus from external validation to internal growth and progress. Concentrate on improving your strength, endurance, and overall fitness levels. Recognize and celebrate your own achievements, regardless of how they compare to others or societal expectations.

5. *Develop Resilience:* Cultivate resilience and a strong sense of self. Remember that criticism and judgment from others often stem from their own insecurities, lack of understanding, or personal biases. Developing a resilient mindset allows you to rise above negativity and maintain confidence in your choices.

6. *Practice Self-Compassion:* Be kind to yourself and practice self-compassion. Accept that not everyone will understand or support your pursuits, but that does not diminish your worth or the value of your journey. Treat yourself with kindness, understanding, and forgiveness as you navigate the challenges and judgments that may arise.

7. *Set Boundaries:* Establish clear boundaries when faced with unsolicited criticism or judgment. Politely but firmly communicate your values and boundaries to those who question or belittle your choices. Remember that you have the right to prioritize your goals and well-being.

8. *Focus on the Positive:* Shift your attention to the positive aspects of female bodybuilding and the benefits it brings to your life. Emphasize the sense of empowerment, discipline, improved health, and personal growth that the sport offers. By focusing on the positive, you can maintain enthusiasm and motivation despite external negativity.

9. *Seek Professional Support:* If criticism and judgment significantly impact your mental and emotional well-being, consider seeking support from a mental health professional. They can provide guidance, strategies, and a safe space to process and navigate the challenges associated with criticism and judgment.

10. *Remember Your Worth:* Above all, remember your worth as an individual. Your value extends far beyond your physical appearance or the opinions of others. Embrace your unique qualities, strengths, and accomplishments. Emphasize self-acceptance, self-love, and self-belief throughout your journey.

Dealing with criticism and judgment is a part of life, particularly for female bodybuilders. By staying true to your goals, surrounding yourself with support, developing resilience, and maintaining a positive mindset, you can navigate these challenges with grace and confidence. Embrace your passion, honor your progress, and remember that the most important validation comes from within yourself.

As we continue through this chapter, we will explore additional aspects of the mental and emotional well-being of female bodybuilders, including motivation, goal setting, overcoming setbacks, and maintaining a healthy mindset.

Finding Support and Building a Community

Finding support and building a community of like-minded individuals is crucial for the mental and emotional well-being of female bodybuilders. Connecting with others who share similar goals, experiences, and challenges can provide invaluable support, motivation, and a sense of belonging. In this section, we will explore strategies for finding support and building a community as a female bodybuilder.

1. Seek Out Local Fitness Facilities: Explore local fitness facilities, gyms, or studios that cater to bodybuilding or strength training. These places often attract individuals with similar interests and goals. Participating in group fitness classes or joining specialized training programs can provide an opportunity to connect with others who share your passion for female bodybuilding.

2. Attend Bodybuilding Events and Competitions: Attend bodybuilding events, competitions, or expos in your area. These gatherings bring together athletes, trainers, and enthusiasts from the bodybuilding community. Engage in conversations, seek advice, and establish connections with individuals who are passionate about the sport.

3. *Join Online Communities:* Utilize social media platforms and online forums to connect with fellow female bodybuilders. Join groups, follow relevant hashtags, and engage in conversations to expand your network and access a wealth of knowledge and support. Online communities provide a platform to share experiences, seek advice, and celebrate accomplishments.

4. *Find a Training Partner:* Consider finding a training partner who shares your passion for female bodybuilding. A training partner can provide support, motivation, and accountability. Collaborating on workouts, sharing tips, and celebrating achievements together can strengthen your bond and enhance your training experience.

5. *Engage in Supportive Conversations:* Actively seek out opportunities to engage in supportive conversations with fellow female bodybuilders. Attend workshops, seminars, or webinars focused on bodybuilding and engage in discussions with participants and experts. Sharing your experiences, challenges, and strategies can foster connections and mutual support.

6. *Connect with Online Coaches or Mentors:* Explore the possibility of working with online coaches or mentors who specialize in female bodybuilding. These professionals can provide personalized guidance, support, and expertise tailored to your specific goals and needs. They can serve as a valuable source of knowledge and motivation throughout your journey.

7. *Participate in Challenges or Transformation Programs:* Engaging in challenges or transformation programs specifically designed for female bodybuilders can create a sense of community and camaraderie. These programs often provide support, resources, and a platform to connect with others who are pursuing similar goals.

8. *Volunteer or Get Involved in Bodybuilding* Organizations: Consider volunteering or getting involved with local bodybuilding organizations or events. By contributing your time and skills, you can become an active member of the bodybuilding community. This involvement allows you to connect with individuals who share your passion and work toward the collective growth and support of the sport.

9. *Share Your Journey and Inspire Others:* Embrace the opportunity to share your own journey and experiences as a female bodybuilder. Use social media, blogs, or other platforms to document your progress, challenges, and triumphs. By sharing your story, you can inspire and motivate others while attracting individuals who resonate with your journey.

10. *Embrace Supportive Relationships:* Cultivate supportive relationships with friends and family who understand and appreciate your dedication to female bodybuilding. Surround yourself with individuals who uplift and encourage you, providing a positive support system outside of the bodybuilding community.

Finding support and building a community as a female bodybuilder can greatly enhance your overall experience and well-being. These connections provide a space for sharing knowledge, seeking advice, celebrating achievements, and finding encouragement during challenging times. By connecting with others who share your passion, you create a supportive network that fuels your motivation and fosters personal growth.

As we progress through this chapter, we will continue exploring various aspects of the mental and emotional well-being of female bodybuilders, including motivation, goal setting, overcoming setbacks, and maintaining a healthy mindset.

Setting Realistic Goals and Maintaining Motivation

Setting realistic goals and maintaining motivation are essential components of the mental and emotional well-being of female bodybuilders. By establishing clear objectives and staying driven throughout your journey, you can experience a sense of purpose, progress, and fulfillment. In this section, we will explore strategies for setting realistic goals and maintaining motivation as a female bodybuilder.

1. Define Your Why: Reflect on the reasons why you have chosen to engage in female bodybuilding. Identify the intrinsic motivations that drive you, such as personal growth, improved health, self-confidence, or a sense of accomplishment. Understanding your deeper motivations will help anchor your goals and keep you motivated during challenging times.

2. Set SMART Goals: Use the SMART goal-setting framework to establish specific, measurable, achievable, relevant, and time-bound goals. Break down your overarching objectives into smaller, actionable steps that are within your reach. This approach helps you stay focused, track progress, and experience a sense of accomplishment along the way.

3. *Prioritize Realistic and Achievable Targets:* While it's important to challenge yourself, setting realistic and attainable goals is crucial for maintaining motivation. Assess your current abilities, consider your lifestyle constraints, and set goals that are within your reach. Gradual progress builds confidence and keeps you motivated to continue pushing forward.

4. *Embrace the Process:* Instead of fixating solely on the end result, embrace the process of female bodybuilding. Recognize that progress takes time and consistent effort. Focus on the daily habits, small improvements, and personal growth that occur throughout your journey. Embracing the process allows you to enjoy the present moment while working towards your long-term goals.

5. *Celebrate Milestones and Achievements:* Take the time to acknowledge and celebrate your milestones and achievements along the way. Whether it's hitting a new personal record, achieving a specific body composition, or mastering a challenging exercise, these moments of success deserve recognition. Celebrating milestones reinforces your progress and boosts motivation.

6. *Find Intrinsic Motivators:* Cultivate intrinsic motivators that ignite your passion and sustain your drive. These can include the enjoyment of the training process, the satisfaction of pushing your limits, or the fulfillment of personal growth. Connecting with the intrinsic aspects of female bodybuilding helps maintain motivation when external factors fluctuate.

7. *Utilize Extrinsic Motivation Strategically:* While intrinsic motivation is powerful, external motivators can also be utilized strategically. Set up rewards or incentives for reaching specific milestones, such as treating yourself to a massage, purchasing new workout attire, or attending a fitness event. These external rewards can provide additional motivation during challenging periods.

8. *Create a Supportive Environment:* Surround yourself with a supportive environment that fosters motivation. Seek out training partners, coaches, or mentors who inspire and challenge you. Engage with a community of like-minded individuals who share similar goals. Being part of a supportive network fuels motivation and provides accountability.

9. *Regularly Assess and Adjust:* Periodically assess your goals, progress, and strategies to ensure they remain aligned with your evolving needs and aspirations. Adjusting your approach based on your experiences and feedback allows for continuous growth and adaptability. Regular reflection and refinement keep your motivation fresh and relevant.

10. Practice Self-Care and Balance: Maintain a healthy balance between your bodybuilding pursuits and other aspects of your life. Prioritize self-care, ensuring you get sufficient rest, engage in activities you enjoy, and maintain fulfilling relationships. Balancing your physical, mental, and emotional well-being contributes to overall motivation and sustainability in the long run.

Setting realistic goals and maintaining motivation as a female bodybuilder require a combination of self-awareness, perseverance, and adaptability. By aligning your goals with your deeper motivations, celebrating milestones, cultivating intrinsic motivation, and creating a supportive environment, you can stay motivated and empowered throughout your bodybuilding journey.

As we continue through this chapter, we will further explore the mental and emotional aspects of female bodybuilding, including strategies for overcoming setbacks, maintaining a healthy mindset, and fostering long-term motivation.

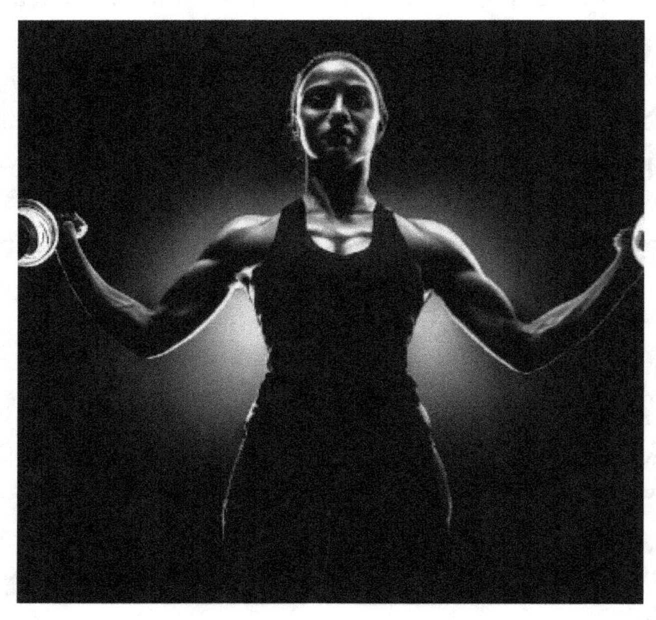

Chapter 6

Female Bodybuilding and Health

Bone Density and Osteoporosis Prevention

Maintaining optimal bone density is crucial for the long-term health and well-being of female bodybuilders. The intense resistance training involved in the sport can have a positive impact on bone health and help prevent conditions like osteoporosis. In this chapter, we will explore the relationship between female bodybuilding and bone density, as well as strategies for osteoporosis prevention.

1. Impact of Resistance Training: The high-intensity resistance training involved in female bodybuilding exerts mechanical stress on the bones, stimulating them to adapt and become stronger. Regular weight-bearing exercises, such as weightlifting, promote bone formation and density, reducing the risk of osteoporosis.

2. Weight-Bearing Exercises: Weight-bearing exercises that involve impact and resistance, such as squats, deadlifts, and lunges, are particularly beneficial for bone health. These exercises put stress on the bones, stimulating them to remodel and become denser. Incorporating a variety of weight-bearing exercises into your training routine can optimize bone health.

3. Progressive Overload: Employing the principle of progressive overload is essential for improving bone density. Gradually increasing the intensity and load of your workouts challenges your bones and prompts them to adapt. This can be achieved through adding resistance, increasing repetitions, or varying exercise difficulty over time.

4. Incorporate Resistance Training: Resistance training, including weightlifting, resistance band exercises, and bodyweight exercises, plays a key role in bone density improvement. Aim to include resistance exercises at least two to three times per week, targeting different muscle groups to promote overall bone health.

5. Proper Form and Technique: Emphasize proper form and technique during weightlifting and resistance exercises. This ensures that the stress is appropriately placed on the bones and muscles, minimizing the risk of injury. If needed, seek guidance from a qualified trainer or coach to learn proper form and technique.

6. *Adequate Calcium and Vitamin D Intake:* Calcium and vitamin D are essential nutrients for bone health. Calcium supports bone mineralization, while vitamin D facilitates calcium absorption. Include calcium-rich foods in your diet, such as dairy products, leafy greens, and fortified plant-based alternatives. Ensure adequate sun exposure or consider a vitamin D supplement if needed.

7. *Balanced Nutrition:* Maintain a balanced diet that supports overall health and provides essential nutrients for bone health. Include a variety of foods rich in vitamins and minerals, such as fruits, vegetables, whole grains, lean proteins, and healthy fats. Proper nutrition helps ensure optimal bone health and supports the body's ability to adapt to training stress.

8. *Avoid Extreme Dieting:* Extreme dieting practices, including severe caloric restriction or excessive exercise without adequate nutrition, can negatively impact bone health. These practices may lead to hormonal imbalances and nutrient deficiencies, compromising bone density. Maintain a well-rounded nutrition plan that supports both your training goals and overall health.

9. *Regular Bone Health Assessments:* Periodically monitor your bone health through bone density assessments, such as dual-energy X-ray absorptiometry

(DEXA) scans. These assessments provide valuable information about your bone mineral density and help detect any potential concerns or areas for improvement.

10. Consult with Healthcare Professionals: If you have concerns about your bone health or are at increased risk of osteoporosis, consult with healthcare professionals, such as your primary care physician or a bone health specialist. They can provide personalized advice, recommend appropriate tests, and offer guidance on optimizing your bone health.

Remember that bone density improvement takes time and consistency. Consistently engaging in weight-bearing exercises, maintaining a balanced diet, and seeking professional guidance when needed can contribute to the long-term health of your bones as a female bodybuilder.

As we progress through this chapter, we will further explore the impact of female bodybuilding on various aspects of health, including cardiovascular health, metabolic health, and overall well-being.

Heart Health and Cardiovascular Benefits

Engaging in female bodybuilding can have significant positive effects on heart health and provide numerous cardiovascular benefits. The combination of resistance training, cardiovascular exercise, and improved body composition contributes to a healthier cardiovascular system. In this chapter, we will explore the relationship between female bodybuilding and heart health, as well as the cardiovascular benefits it offers.

1. Strengthens the Heart Muscle: Regular resistance training, such as weightlifting, increases the workload on the heart, strengthening the cardiac muscle. As you progressively challenge your muscles, your heart adapts by becoming more efficient at pumping blood, leading to improved overall cardiovascular function.

2. Improves Cardiovascular Endurance: Incorporating cardiovascular exercises, such as running, cycling, or swimming, into your training regimen enhances cardiovascular endurance. These exercises increase your heart rate and respiratory rate, stimulating the cardiovascular system and improving its efficiency over time.

3. Reduces Risk Factors: Female bodybuilding can help reduce several risk factors associated with cardiovascular diseases, such as high blood pressure, elevated cholesterol levels, and obesity. Regular exercise, combined with a balanced diet and a healthy lifestyle, helps manage these risk factors and promotes better heart health.

4. Enhances Blood Circulation: Engaging in physical activity, including resistance training and cardiovascular exercises, improves blood circulation throughout the body. This enhanced circulation ensures that oxygen and nutrients are delivered efficiently to the tissues, including the heart muscle itself.

5. Supports Weight Management: Female bodybuilding, with its focus on strength training and building lean muscle mass, contributes to improved body composition. Increased muscle mass boosts the body's metabolic rate, helping to maintain a healthy weight or promote weight loss. Maintaining a healthy weight reduces the strain on the cardiovascular system, improving heart health.

6. Reduces Inflammation and Oxidative Stress: Regular exercise, including female bodybuilding, helps reduce chronic inflammation and oxidative stress in the body. These two factors play a significant role in the development of cardiovascular diseases. By reducing inflammation and oxidative stress, female bodybuilding promotes better heart health.

7. *Enhances Vascular Health:* Resistance training and cardiovascular exercise improve the health and function of blood vessels, promoting their elasticity and reducing the risk of atherosclerosis (hardening of the arteries). This enhanced vascular health supports optimal blood flow and reduces the risk of heart-related complications.

8. *Lowers Resting Heart Rate:* Engaging in regular exercise, including female bodybuilding, can lower resting heart rate over time. A lower resting heart rate indicates that the heart is functioning efficiently and does not have to work as hard during periods of rest, resulting in improved cardiovascular health.

9. *Improves Lipid Profile:* Exercise, including resistance training, has been shown to positively impact lipid profiles by increasing levels of "good" cholesterol (HDL cholesterol) and reducing levels of "bad" cholesterol (LDL cholesterol) and triglycerides. This favorable lipid profile decreases the risk of developing cardiovascular diseases.

10. *Stress Reduction:* Regular exercise, including female bodybuilding, helps reduce stress levels. High levels of stress can contribute to cardiovascular problems, so managing stress through exercise can have a positive impact on heart health.

It is important to note that before starting any exercise program, including female bodybuilding, it is advisable to consult with your healthcare provider, especially if you have pre-existing cardiovascular conditions or concerns. They can provide personalized guidance and recommendations based on your individual health status.

By engaging in female bodybuilding and incorporating a well-rounded exercise regimen, you can experience significant improvements in heart health and overall cardiovascular function. The combination of resistance training, cardiovascular exercise, and healthy lifestyle practices offers substantial benefits for the cardiovascular system.

As we continue through this chapter, we will further explore the impact of female bodybuilding on various aspects of health, including metabolic health, mental well-being, and overall physical well-being.

Hormonal Balance and Menstrual Health

Female bodybuilding can have an impact on hormonal balance and menstrual health. The rigorous training and dietary practices involved in the sport may affect hormonal regulation, potentially influencing the menstrual cycle. In this chapter, we will explore the relationship between female bodybuilding and hormonal balance, as well as strategies for maintaining healthy menstrual function.

1. Understanding Hormonal Changes: Intense training and low body fat levels associated with female bodybuilding can lead to hormonal changes. These changes may include alterations in levels of estrogen, progesterone, and other hormones involved in the menstrual cycle. Understanding and monitoring these changes are important for maintaining overall hormonal balance.

2. Energy Balance and Menstrual Health: Maintaining an appropriate energy balance is crucial for preserving menstrual health. Extreme caloric restriction or excessive energy expenditure without adequate nutrition can disrupt the delicate hormonal balance and lead to irregular or absent menstrual cycles. It is important to strike a balance between energy expenditure and nutrition to support healthy menstrual function.

3. Nourishing Nutrition: Proper nutrition plays a vital role in supporting hormonal balance and menstrual health. Consuming a well-rounded diet that includes an adequate intake of macronutrients, micronutrients, and essential fatty acids is important. Prioritize nutrient-dense foods, such as fruits, vegetables, whole grains, lean proteins, and healthy fats, to support overall hormonal function.

4. Sufficient Caloric Intake: Ensuring sufficient caloric intake is crucial for maintaining menstrual health. Women engaged in female bodybuilding may have higher caloric needs due to increased training intensity and muscle mass. Adequate caloric intake supports the energy requirements of the menstrual cycle and helps prevent disruptions to hormonal balance.

5. Balanced Exercise Routine: Balancing exercise intensity and volume is important for preserving hormonal balance. Excessive exercise, particularly when combined with low body fat levels, can lead to hormonal imbalances and menstrual irregularities. Strive for a balanced exercise routine that includes both resistance training and cardiovascular exercise while allowing sufficient rest and recovery.

6. Prioritize Rest and Recovery: Rest and recovery are essential for maintaining hormonal balance and menstrual health. Adequate sleep, stress management, and incorporating rest days into your training regimen are important factors in supporting healthy hormonal function. Overtraining and chronic stress can negatively impact the menstrual cycle.

7. Individualize Training and Nutrition: Recognize that every woman's body is unique, and what works for one may not work for another. It is crucial to individualize training and nutrition approaches based on your own needs, goals, and menstrual patterns. Pay attention to your body's signals and adjust your training and nutrition plan accordingly.

8. Consult with Healthcare Professionals: If you experience significant disruptions to your menstrual cycle or have concerns about hormonal balance, it is advisable to consult with healthcare professionals, such as a gynecologist or endocrinologist who specializes in women's health. They can provide personalized advice, assess your hormonal status, and offer appropriate interventions if needed.

9. Monitor Menstrual Function: Keep track of your menstrual cycle, noting any changes or irregularities.

Maintaining a menstrual diary can help you identify patterns or potential disruptions. If you notice significant changes or irregularities, consult with a healthcare professional to assess and address any underlying issues.

10. Strive for Overall Balance: Strive for balance in all aspects of your life, including training, nutrition, rest, and stress management. Aim for a holistic approach to health that supports hormonal balance and overall well-being. Remember that achieving and maintaining hormonal balance is a dynamic process that may require ongoing adjustments.

Maintaining hormonal balance and menstrual health is important for the overall well-being of female bodybuilders. By adopting a balanced approach to training, nutrition, rest, and self-care, you can support healthy hormonal function and preserve menstrual health. Prioritizing individualized care and seeking professional guidance when needed can further optimize hormonal balance.

As we continue through this chapter, we will further explore the impact of female bodybuilding on various aspects of health, including metabolic health, mental well-being, and overall physical well-being.

Addressing Potential Risks and Injuries

While female bodybuilding offers numerous health benefits, it is important to be aware of potential risks and injuries associated with the sport. Understanding these risks and taking preventive measures can help minimize the likelihood of injury and ensure a safe and sustainable bodybuilding journey. In this chapter, we will explore common risks and injuries in female bodybuilding and strategies for addressing them.

1. Muscle Strains and Tears: The intense training involved in bodybuilding can put stress on muscles, increasing the risk of strains and tears. Proper warm-up and cool-down routines, adequate stretching, and gradually increasing the intensity of exercises can help prevent muscle injuries. Pay attention to proper form and technique during training to reduce the risk of strain or tear.

2. Joint and Tendon Issues: Repetitive motions and heavy loads can lead to joint and tendon issues, such as tendinitis or joint inflammation. Incorporating exercises that strengthen supporting muscles around joints, using proper lifting techniques, and giving ample rest and recovery to the affected areas can help reduce the risk of joint and tendon injuries.

3. Overuse Injuries: Overtraining or excessive repetition of certain movements can lead to overuse injuries, such as stress fractures or tendinopathies. It is important to balance training intensity and volume, allowing sufficient rest and recovery. Varying your exercises, cross-training, and incorporating rest days into your training schedule can help prevent overuse injuries.

4. Bone Health Concerns: While female bodybuilding can improve bone density, excessive training combined with inadequate nutrition may lead to bone-related issues. Ensure a balanced diet that provides sufficient nutrients for bone health, including calcium, vitamin D, and other essential minerals. Regular bone health assessments and consulting with healthcare professionals can help address any concerns.

5. Hormonal Imbalances: Intense training and low body fat levels in female bodybuilding can potentially lead to hormonal imbalances. Monitoring menstrual health, ensuring adequate nutrition and caloric intake, and seeking professional guidance when needed can help address and manage hormonal imbalances.

6. Psychological Well-being: The intense focus on physique and competition in bodybuilding can sometimes impact psychological well-being. It is important to maintain a healthy mindset, prioritize self-care, and seek support from a mental health professional if needed. Building a balanced lifestyle that includes interests beyond bodybuilding can contribute to overall psychological well-being.

7. *Cardiovascular Stress:* While cardiovascular exercise offers benefits, excessive cardio combined with high-intensity resistance training can potentially stress the cardiovascular system. Monitoring training intensity, incorporating adequate recovery periods, and consulting with healthcare professionals can help manage cardiovascular stress.

8. *Nutritional Deficiencies:* Strict dietary practices or extreme caloric restriction can lead to nutritional deficiencies, compromising overall health and performance. Prioritize a well-rounded, nutrient-dense diet that supports your training and consult with a registered dietitian or nutritionist to ensure optimal nutrition.

9. *Body Image Concerns:* Bodybuilding's emphasis on physique can sometimes contribute to body image concerns or disordered eating behaviors. Promote a healthy body image by focusing on overall well-being, setting realistic goals, and seeking support from professionals or support groups if needed.

10. Injury Prevention Strategies: Incorporating proper warm-up and cool-down routines, following a structured training program, using correct lifting techniques, and listening to your body's signals are essential for injury prevention. Consulting with certified trainers or coaches knowledgeable in bodybuilding can help ensure safe and effective training practices.

By understanding and addressing potential risks and injuries in female bodybuilding, you can enjoy the sport while prioritizing your health and well-being. Employing preventive measures, seeking professional guidance when needed, and maintaining a balanced approach to training, nutrition, and recovery can support a safe and sustainable bodybuilding journey.

As we progress through this chapter, we will further explore the impact of female bodybuilding on various aspects of health, including metabolic health, mental well-being, and overall physical well-being.

Chapter 7

The Future of Female Bodybuilding

Breaking Barriers and Expanding Opportunities

Female bodybuilding has come a long way, and its future holds exciting possibilities for breaking barriers and expanding opportunities for women in the sport. Over the years, female bodybuilders have shattered stereotypes, challenged societal norms, and gained recognition for their dedication, athleticism, and aesthetic achievements. In this chapter, we will explore the evolving landscape of female bodybuilding and the potential for growth and inclusivity.

1. Increased Visibility and Recognition: Female bodybuilders have gained increased visibility and recognition within the fitness industry and beyond. Through competitions, social media platforms, documentaries, and media coverage, their accomplishments and stories are being shared, highlighting the dedication, discipline, and athleticism involved in the sport.

2. Challenging Gender Stereotypes: Female bodybuilding has played a significant role in challenging traditional gender stereotypes that associate muscularity and strength primarily with men. Women in bodybuilding continue to redefine beauty standards and showcase the power and strength that can be achieved through dedicated training and discipline.

3. Diversity and Inclusivity: The future of female bodybuilding holds great potential for embracing diversity and inclusivity. As the sport continues to grow, it is important to celebrate and support bodybuilders from various backgrounds, ethnicities, body types, and age groups. Embracing diversity enhances the richness and inclusiveness of the bodybuilding community.

4. Expanding Categories and Divisions: Female bodybuilding competitions have evolved to include a broader range of categories and divisions, catering to different goals, preferences, and body types. This expansion provides more opportunities for women to participate and compete in a way that aligns with their individual strengths and aspirations.

5. Empowering and Inspiring Others: Female bodybuilders serve as powerful role models, inspiring others to pursue their fitness goals, overcome obstacles, and prioritize their health and well-being. The future of female bodybuilding holds the potential for even greater empowerment, creating a ripple effect of positive change and motivation among women of all ages and backgrounds.

6. *Advocating for Equality:* Female bodybuilding has been at the forefront of advocating for equality in the fitness industry. As the sport continues to evolve, there is an opportunity to push for equal recognition, resources, and opportunities for female athletes. Advocating for equal pay, sponsorship opportunities, and media representation can further enhance the future of female bodybuilding.

7. *Embracing Wellness and Overall Health:* The future of female bodybuilding may also witness a greater emphasis on overall wellness and health. Bodybuilders are increasingly focusing on holistic well-being, including mental health, balanced nutrition, and sustainable training practices. This shift promotes a healthier and more balanced approach to the sport.

8. *Leveraging Technology and Education:* Technology and educational resources play a vital role in shaping the future of female bodybuilding. Online platforms, fitness apps, and educational content can provide valuable information, training programs, and community support for aspiring female bodybuilders. Utilizing these tools can enhance accessibility and foster knowledge-sharing among athletes worldwide.

9. *Collaboration and Support:* Collaboration and support within the female bodybuilding community are essential for its future growth and success. Athletes, trainers, coaches, and organizations can work together to share best practices, mentorship programs, and resources, creating a supportive network that fosters development and camaraderie.

10. *Inspiring Body Positivity:* The future of female bodybuilding holds the potential to inspire body positivity and self-acceptance. By promoting diverse body types, celebrating individual achievements, and focusing on overall health and well-being, female bodybuilders can help redefine beauty standards and foster a culture of self-love and acceptance.

The future of female bodybuilding is bright and promising, with opportunities to break barriers, expand inclusivity, and inspire generations to come. As the sport evolves, embracing diversity, advocating for equality, and prioritizing overall health and well-being will shape a future that empowers women and celebrates their achievements in the world of bodybuilding.

Inspiring the Next Generation of Female Bodybuilders

One of the most exciting aspects of the future of female bodybuilding is the opportunity to inspire and empower the next generation of female bodybuilders. As women continue to push boundaries and redefine what is possible in the sport, they have the ability to inspire young girls and women to pursue their own passions, challenge societal norms, and embrace their inner strength. In this chapter, we will explore strategies for inspiring and nurturing the next generation of female bodybuilders.

1. Visibility and Representation: Increasing visibility and representation of female bodybuilders is crucial for inspiring the next generation. Through social media, competitions, documentaries, and media features, showcasing diverse and relatable role models allows young girls and women to see themselves reflected in the sport. Highlighting the stories, achievements, and journeys of female bodybuilders can inspire others to pursue their own athletic aspirations.

2. Mentorship and Guidance: Establishing mentorship programs and providing guidance to young aspiring female bodybuilders can be immensely impactful. Experienced athletes, trainers, and coaches can offer support, knowledge, and encouragement to help navigate the challenges and obstacles in the sport. Mentorship programs can provide guidance on training, nutrition, competition preparation, and overall well-being.

3. *Education and Resources:* Providing educational resources specifically tailored to young female bodybuilders is essential. This includes age-appropriate information on training techniques, nutrition, injury prevention, and the importance of overall health. Developing accessible and engaging educational materials, such as books, articles, videos, and workshops, can equip aspiring female bodybuilders with the knowledge they need to succeed.

4. *Fostering a Positive and Supportive Environment:* Creating a positive and supportive environment is crucial for nurturing the next generation of female bodybuilders. Encouraging teamwork, collaboration, and sportsmanship helps foster camaraderie and a sense of community among young athletes. Promoting a culture of inclusivity, acceptance, and support ensures that all aspiring female bodybuilders feel welcome and empowered.

5. *Emphasizing the Journey and Personal Growth:* Inspiring the next generation of female bodybuilders involves highlighting the journey and personal growth that comes with the sport. Encouraging young athletes to focus on their progress, resilience, and dedication rather than solely on external appearances or competition outcomes promotes a healthy mindset and long-term sustainability in the sport.

6. *Promoting Body Positivity and Self-Acceptance:* Instilling body positivity and self-acceptance is crucial for the mental and emotional well-being of young female bodybuilders. Emphasizing that beauty comes in diverse forms and celebrating individual strengths and unique qualities helps young athletes develop a positive body image. Encouraging self-care, self-love, and acceptance of one's own body fosters a healthy relationship with the sport.

7. *Encouraging Balanced Development:* It is important to encourage young female bodybuilders to develop a well-rounded approach to their athletic journey. Balancing training with other interests, maintaining academic commitments, and nurturing social relationships contributes to their overall development and well-being. Encouraging a healthy work-life balance supports long-term success and fulfillment.

8. *Empowering Leadership Skills:* Empowering young female bodybuilders with leadership skills is essential for their growth and future impact in the sport.

Encouraging them to take on leadership roles within their training groups, clubs, or communities fosters confidence, resilience, and a sense of responsibility. Leadership skills empower young athletes to become advocates for themselves and the sport.

9. ***Celebrating Achievements:*** Celebrating the achievements of young female bodybuilders, no matter how big or small, is important for their motivation and self-belief. Recognizing their progress, effort, and dedication helps build their confidence and reinforces the value of hard work and perseverance. Creating platforms or events to showcase and celebrate the accomplishments of young athletes can inspire others and create a supportive community.

10. ***Encouraging Positive Role Models:*** Encouraging young female bodybuilders to seek positive role models both within and outside the sport can broaden their perspective and inspire them in various aspects of their lives. Highlighting accomplished female athletes, professionals, and trailblazers from diverse fields encourages young athletes to dream big, set ambitious goals, and pursue excellence.

By inspiring and nurturing the next generation of female bodybuilders, we can create a legacy of empowered and confident women who continue to push boundaries, challenge stereotypes, and achieve greatness in the sport. The future holds tremendous potential for young girls and women to embrace their inner strength, pursue their passions, and make a lasting impact on the world of female bodybuilding.

As we conclude this book, we hope that the information and insights shared have provided valuable guidance and inspiration to both current and aspiring female bodybuilders. The future is bright, and it is in the hands of the next generation to continue the legacy of female empowerment in the world of bodybuilding.

Shifting Perspectives and Changing Stereotypes

The future of female bodybuilding holds the potential to shift perspectives and challenge the stereotypes that have long surrounded the sport. As women continue to excel in bodybuilding, breaking barriers and achieving remarkable feats of strength and athleticism, society's perception of female bodybuilders is evolving. In this chapter, we will explore the power of female bodybuilders in shifting perspectives and changing stereotypes.

1. Redefining Beauty Standards: Female bodybuilders play a pivotal role in redefining beauty standards and challenging conventional notions of femininity. By showcasing their muscular physiques, dedication, and hard work, they demonstrate that strength and athleticism can be empowering and beautiful. Their presence challenges the narrow definition of beauty and encourages a more inclusive and diverse perspective.

2. Promoting Body Positivity: Female bodybuilders are powerful advocates for body positivity. By embracing and celebrating their muscular bodies, they inspire others to appreciate and accept diverse body types. Their confidence and self-acceptance serve as a powerful reminder that beauty comes in many forms, fostering a culture of body positivity and self-love.

3. *Breaking Gender Stereotypes:* Female bodybuilders break down gender stereotypes by showcasing their strength and physical capabilities. They challenge the notion that women are inherently weaker or less suited for intense physical pursuits. By defying these stereotypes, female bodybuilders inspire others to challenge societal norms and embrace their own strengths and abilities.

4. *Inspiring Empowerment and Confidence:* The dedication and discipline required in female bodybuilding inspire empowerment and confidence. Female bodybuilders demonstrate that through hard work and determination, women can achieve extraordinary feats, both inside and outside the gym. Their stories and achievements motivate others to pursue their own goals with courage and self-belief.

5. *Advocating for Equality:* Female bodybuilders are at the forefront of advocating for equality within the fitness industry. They work to ensure equal recognition, opportunities, and resources for female athletes. By raising their voices and advocating for change, they challenge gender disparities and pave the way for a more inclusive and equitable future.

6. *Educating and Debunking Myths:* Female bodybuilders play a crucial role in educating others about the realities of the sport and debunking common myths and misconceptions. By sharing their knowledge and experiences, they dispel stereotypes surrounding female bodybuilding, such as the belief that it leads to a "masculine" appearance or compromises femininity. Their education efforts contribute to a better understanding of the sport and its benefits.

7. *Empowering Other Women:* Female bodybuilders inspire and empower other women to pursue their own fitness goals and embrace strength training. They serve as role models, encouraging women to challenge their limits, embrace their physical power, and prioritize their health and well-being. Their influence extends beyond the gym, empowering women to embrace their strength in all aspects of life.

8. *Cultivating a Supportive Community:* Female bodybuilders foster a supportive community that encourages camaraderie, respect, and mutual support. By building connections and networks, they create spaces where women feel encouraged, accepted, and celebrated for their achievements. This supportive community empowers female bodybuilders to thrive and inspires others to join the movement.

9. *Inspiring Younger Generations:* Female bodybuilders have the power to inspire younger generations to challenge stereotypes and embrace their unique strengths. By serving as role models for young girls, they demonstrate that success and fulfillment come from pursuing one's passions, breaking boundaries, and defying societal expectations. Their influence helps shape a more inclusive and empowered future.

10. *Contributing to Cultural Change:* Through their presence and achievements, female bodybuilders contribute to a broader cultural change. They challenge traditional gender roles, ignite conversations about body image and strength, and push for a more inclusive and accepting society. Their impact extends beyond the confines of the sport, shaping societal perceptions and encouraging a more diverse and inclusive understanding of strength and beauty.

The future of female bodybuilding holds immense potential to shift perspectives and change stereotypes. Female bodybuilders are powerful agents of change, inspiring empowerment, challenging norms, and promoting inclusivity. As their influence continues to grow, the impact they make in reshaping societal perceptions will create a more accepting and supportive environment for women in bodybuilding and beyond.

Conclusion

"Female Bodybuilding Myths and Facts: Debunking the Misconceptions About This Sport" has explored the multifaceted world of female bodybuilding, shedding light on the truths, dispelling myths, and challenging stereotypes surrounding this empowering sport. Throughout this book, we have delved into various aspects of female bodybuilding, including its evolution, benefits, nutritional considerations, common misconceptions, training strategies, and the impact on mental and physical well-being. We have also explored the future of female bodybuilding, envisioning a future marked by inclusivity, empowerment, and a shift in societal perspectives.

In our exploration, we have witnessed the remarkable dedication, resilience, and strength of female bodybuilders who have defied expectations and shattered barriers. They have emerged as role models, inspiring others to embrace their inner power, challenge societal norms, and pursue their fitness goals with determination and confidence. By sharing their stories, accomplishments, and knowledge, female bodybuilders have played a crucial role in expanding opportunities, fostering inclusivity, and reshaping the perception of beauty and strength.

We have debunked prevalent myths and misconceptions surrounding female bodybuilding, challenging the notion that it leads to a masculine appearance, compromises femininity, or is solely for professional athletes. Instead, we have highlighted the myriad benefits, including enhanced physical fitness, improved cardiovascular health, increased bone density, mental resilience, and the cultivation of self-esteem and body positivity.

Through this journey, we have emphasized the importance of balanced nutrition, proper training techniques, rest and recovery, and individualized approaches tailored to each woman's goals and needs. We have explored the integral role of education, mentorship, and support in nurturing the next generation of female bodybuilders, inspiring them to pursue their passions, challenge stereotypes, and foster a sense of empowerment and self-acceptance.

The future of female bodybuilding holds great promise. It is a future that embraces diversity, advocates for equality, and cultivates a supportive and inclusive community. As female bodybuilders continue to break barriers, change stereotypes, and inspire others, they pave the way for a future where strength, determination, and resilience are celebrated in all their forms.

In closing, "Female Bodybuilding Myths and Facts: Debunking the Misconceptions About This Sport" encourages readers to embrace the strength within themselves, challenge societal norms, and pursue their fitness goals with passion and dedication. By dispelling myths, fostering education, and promoting a culture of inclusivity, we can create a future where female bodybuilding is recognized as a testament to the power, beauty, and incredible potential of women in the world of sports and beyond.

As we embark on our own journeys, let us carry the lessons learned from this book—acceptance, perseverance, and the courage to challenge misconceptions—into all aspects of our lives. May we celebrate the achievements of female bodybuilders, support one another in our pursuits, and continue to reshape the narrative surrounding female strength and athleticism.

The future of female bodybuilding is bright, and it is in our collective power to ensure that it continues to evolve, inspire, and empower generations to come.